OSTEOPOROSIS OASIS

Therapies For Stronger Bones And Joint Support

Strengthen Bones And Joints With Innovative Therapies That Address Osteoporosis And Promote Musculoskeletal Well-Being

DR. BRIDGET PROMISE

CHAPTER ONE

Introduction

Osteoporosis, a disorder characterized by weakening and brittle bones, is a major public health problem affecting millions of individuals worldwide. As bone density and strength decrease, the risk of fractures and injuries rises, having a significant effect on general health and well-being.

In this discussion, we will look at the notion of osteoporosis, how it affects bone health, the variables that lead to its development, and effective preventative techniques.

Understanding Osteoporosis

Osteoporosis is a skeletal condition in which bone tissue deteriorates and bone density decreases.

Bones are dynamic structures that are continually renewing themselves, replacing old bone with new bone. However, in people with osteoporosis, this equilibrium is altered, making them more vulnerable to fractures and breaks.

Bone is a living tissue made up of a protein matrix (mainly collagen) and minerals like calcium and phosphorus. Bone strength and density are determined by their appropriate balance of components. When bone density declines, it becomes porous and weak, making it more susceptible to fractures even with mild impact.

Impact On Bone Health

Osteoporosis has a significant influence on bone health, going beyond the increased risk of fractures. While fractures are a major problem, especially in weight-bearing bones such as the hip, spine, and wrist, the total structural integrity of the skeletal system is jeopardized.

One of the most common outcomes of osteoporosis is a loss of height and stooped posture caused by compression fractures in the spine. Vertebral fractures may develop without any obvious damage and cause persistent discomfort, limited mobility, and a worse quality of life.

Furthermore, fractures in the hip and other major bones may lead to serious problems, such as disability and an increased risk of death, particularly in older persons.

Furthermore, osteoporosis may have a significant influence on everyday activities, causing limits in mobility and functioning. Fear of fractures may cause a decrease in physical activity, perpetuating a cycle of decreased bone density, muscular weakness, and an increased chance of falling.

CHAPTER TWO

Risk Factors And Prevention Strategy

Several variables influence the development of osteoporosis, and recognizing these risk factors is critical for successful prevention. Some risk factors, such as age, gender, and heredity, are beyond an individual's control, whilst others may be changed by lifestyle choices.

1. Age and gender: Osteoporosis is more common in elderly persons since bone density gradually declines with age. Women, particularly those who have had

menopause, are at a greater risk owing to hormonal changes that influence bone remodeling.

2. Genetics: Family history influences an individual's vulnerability to osteoporosis. If a close family member suffers fractures caused by osteoporosis, there may be a hereditary predisposition that raises the risk.

3. Hormonal Changes: Hormonal variables, notably a drop in estrogen levels in postmenopausal women, may contribute to bone loss. Men's testosterone levels also fall as they age, which may influence bone density.

4. Nutrition and Calcium consumption: Insufficient calcium and vitamin D consumption may harm bone health. Calcium is an essential element for bone strength, and a lack may hasten bone loss.

5. Physical Activity: Sedentary lifestyles lead to bone weakness and muscular atrophy. Weight-bearing workouts and strength training are essential for maintaining bone density and skeletal health.

6. Smoking and heavy alcohol intake are bad for bone health. Both drugs may impair the body's

capacity to absorb calcium, thus impacting bone rebuilding.

7. Medical diseases and Medications: Certain medical diseases, such as rheumatoid arthritis and hormone imbalances, may exacerbate osteoporosis. Furthermore, chronic use of some drugs, such as corticosteroids, may weaken bones.

Osteoporosis prevention techniques include lifestyle changes as well as medical treatments. Adequate calcium and vitamin D consumption, either via food or supplements, is needed for bone health. Regular weight-bearing workouts, such as walking, running, and resistance training, help to strengthen bones and improve general health.

Quitting smoking and reducing alcohol use are important lifestyle decisions for avoiding osteoporosis. Smoking quitting not only helps the respiratory system, but it also improves bone health. Alcohol consumption should be restricted since it might interfere with bone metabolism.

Regular bone density examinations, particularly for those at greater risk, may help with early identification and management. Those who are at high risk of fractures may benefit from medical therapies, such as prescription drugs that enhance bone density.

Osteoporosis is a complicated and serious disorder that affects bone health and general well-being. As we age, the need to take proactive steps to preserve bone density and strength becomes more apparent. Understanding the variables that contribute to osteoporosis and adopting effective preventative methods, both via lifestyle changes and medicinal therapies, is critical for improving bone health and lowering the risk of fracture.

Individuals may improve their quality of life and retain their independence as they age by addressing their bone health holistically.

Osteoporosis, a prevalent skeletal illness marked by poor bone density and eroding bone tissue, is a major concern in contemporary healthcare. Addressing this problem requires a thorough grasp of diagnostic techniques, medical treatments, pharmacological therapies, and nutritional support for bone health.

Diagnostic Approaches

An accurate diagnosis is the basis of successful osteoporosis care. Healthcare practitioners use a variety of diagnostic methods to evaluate bone health and identify persons at risk. Dual-energy X-ray absorptiometry (DXA) scans, the gold standard for bone density testing, give exact measurements of bone mineral density (BMD). DXA scans can diagnose osteoporosis and estimate fracture risk. Another diagnostic strategy is to include clinical risk variables such as age, gender, family history, and lifestyle. Combining DXA data with clinical risk factors improves diagnostic accuracy and helps choose the best course of action.

Bone turnover markers, or biochemical indicators in blood and urine that indicate bone remodeling activity, provide further information on bone health. High levels of these markers may indicate greater bone resorption and a higher risk of fracture. While bone turnover indicators are not employed as solo diagnostic tools, they provide useful information when combined with other diagnostic techniques.

CHAPTER THREE

Medical Treatment For Osteoporosis

Once diagnosed, the emphasis changes to medical therapies to manage osteoporosis and prevent fractures. Pharmacological therapies and lifestyle changes play critical roles in the entire therapy regimen.

Pharmacological Interventions

Several types of medications are available to treat osteoporosis and improve bone health. Bisphosphonates, including alendronate and risedronate, are among the most widely prescribed medications. They inhibit bone resorption by targeting osteoclasts, the cells that break down bone tissue. Denosumab, a monoclonal antibody, is another option that inhibits osteoclast activity, thereby slowing bone loss.

Selective estrogen receptor modulators (SERMs), such as raloxifene, mimic the effects of estrogen in specific tissues, increasing bone density while lowering the risk of fracture. Hormone therapy, particularly in postmenopausal women, may be considered to counteract the decline in estrogen levels caused by bone loss.

Teriparatide and abaloparatide, both forms of parathyroid hormone, promote bone formation and are used in situations where other medications may not be appropriate or effective. These medications are usually given as injections and are reserved for severe osteoporosis cases.

Calcium and vitamin D supplements are frequently recommended in conjunction with pharmacological interventions to maintain optimal bone health. Calcium is an essential component of bone structure, and vitamin D promotes calcium absorption. Both nutrients must be present at adequate levels for osteoporosis medications to be effective.

Nutritional Support For Bone Health

In addition to medications, nutritional support is essential for managing osteoporosis and promoting overall bone health. Adequate calcium, vitamin D, and other essential nutrients promote bone strength and density.

Calcium is an essential mineral for bone health, and a lack can cause increased bone fragility. Dairy products, leafy green vegetables, and fortified foods are excellent dietary sources of calcium. However, achieving the recommended daily intake through diet alone can be challenging, prompting the need for calcium supplements in some cases.

Vitamin D is essential for calcium absorption, and insufficient levels can compromise bone health. Exposure to sunlight triggers vitamin D synthesis in the skin, but dietary sources and supplements may be necessary, especially in regions with limited sunlight or for individuals with restricted sun exposure.

Maintaining an overall healthy diet is crucial for supporting bone health. Adequate protein intake is essential, as proteins form the structural framework of bones. Additionally, micronutrients such as magnesium, phosphorus, vitamin K, and vitamin C contribute to bone metabolism and maintenance.

Collaboration between healthcare professionals and nutritionists is vital to tailor dietary recommendations to individual needs. The integration of nutritional support with medical treatments enhances the comprehensive approach to osteoporosis management.

In conclusion, addressing osteoporosis involves a multi-faceted approach encompassing diagnostic measures, medical treatments, pharmacological interventions, and nutritional support. Accurate diagnosis through tools like DXA scans and consideration of clinical risk factors lays the groundwork for effective intervention. Pharmacological options, including bisphosphonates, SERMs, and parathyroid hormone analogs, offer diverse strategies for managing bone health. Nutritional support, particularly through adequate calcium and vitamin D intake, complements medical interventions and contributes to overall bone strength. A holistic approach that combines diagnostic precision, medical expertise, and nutritional guidance is crucial for mitigating the impact of osteoporosis on individuals' quality of life.

Exercise Regimens For Stronger Bones

Bones play a crucial role in providing structural support, protecting vital organs, and facilitating movement. As we age, maintaining bone health becomes increasingly important to prevent conditions like osteoporosis and fractures. Incorporating targeted exercise regimens into your routine is a proactive approach to strengthen bones and improve overall skeletal health.

Regular weight-bearing exercises are particularly effective in promoting bone strength. Weight-bearing exercises involve activities that force you to work against gravity, stimulating bone formation and density. Examples of such exercises include walking, jogging, hiking, and dancing. These activities engage various muscle groups and bones, promoting bone remodeling and growth.

In addition to weight-bearing exercises, resistance training is beneficial for bone health. Strength training with weights, resistance bands, or body weight helps build muscle mass, which, in turn, supports and strengthens bones. Focus on compound exercises such as squats, lunges, and deadlifts to target multiple muscle groups and enhance bone density.

CHAPTER FOUR

Alternative Therapies: A Holistic Approach

Beyond standard exercise regimes, alternative medicines provide a comprehensive approach to boosting bone health. While these therapies may not replace traditional methods, they can complement and enhance the overall well-being of your skeletal system.

One such alternative therapy is yoga. Yoga combines gentle stretching, balance, and weight-bearing poses, making it an excellent choice for improving bone density. Certain yoga poses, like tree pose and warrior poses, engage the lower body, hips, and spine, promoting flexibility and strength. The mindful and meditative aspects of yoga also contribute to stress reduction, positively impacting overall health and bone density.

Another alternative therapy gaining recognition for bone health is acupuncture. Rooted in traditional Chinese medicine, acupuncture involves the insertion of thin needles into specific points on the body to stimulate energy flow. Some studies suggest that acupuncture may help reduce pain associated with bone conditions and contribute to better overall bone health.

Lifestyle Changes For Bone Density

In addition to targeted exercises and alternative therapies, making certain lifestyle changes can significantly impact bone density. Proper nutrition, including an adequate intake of calcium and vitamin D, is fundamental for maintaining strong bones.

Calcium is a crucial mineral for bone structure, and vitamin D helps the body absorb calcium efficiently.

Include dairy products, leafy greens, and fortified foods in your diet to ensure an ample supply of calcium. Sun exposure is an excellent natural source of vitamin D, but supplements may be required, particularly for those who receive little sun exposure. Consult a healthcare practitioner to discover the best complement for your specific requirements.

Avoiding tobacco and limiting alcohol consumption is also vital for bone health. Smoking has been linked to a decrease in bone density, while excessive alcohol intake can interfere with the body's ability to absorb essential nutrients for bone health. Adopting a smoke-free lifestyle and regulating alcohol use contribute significantly to bone density and general well-being.

Maintaining a healthy body weight is another lifestyle element that affects bone health. Both underweight and obesity may severely influence bone density.

Strive for a balanced diet and frequent exercise to reach and maintain a healthy weight, providing optimum support for your bones.

Joint Support And Mobility Enhancement

Maintaining joint health is an integral part of overall bone health, as joints and bones work in tandem to facilitate movement. Joint support and mobility enhancement strategies can help prevent injuries, reduce stiffness, and contribute to overall skeletal well-being.

Incorporating joint-friendly exercises is essential for preserving joint health. Low-impact activities such as swimming, cycling, and elliptical training provide cardiovascular benefits without placing excessive stress on the joints. These exercises enhance mobility, reduce inflammation, and contribute to joint flexibility.

Another aspect of joint support is the use of supplements known to promote joint health. Glucosamine and chondroitin are commonly used supplements believed to support joint structure and function. These substances are naturally found in cartilage and may help alleviate joint pain and stiffness. As with any supplement, it's advisable to consult with a healthcare professional before incorporating them into your routine.

Maintaining proper posture is crucial for joint support, particularly in the spine and hips. Poor posture can cause misalignment, increasing stress on joints and bones. Exercises that focus on core strength and flexibility can help you maintain a healthy posture and reduce your risk of joint issues.

To summarize, a comprehensive approach to bone health combines targeted exercise regimens, alternative therapies, lifestyle changes, and joint support strategies. By incorporating these elements into your daily routine, you can strengthen your bones, improve overall skeletal health, and improve your quality of life. Remember to consult with a healthcare professional before making any significant changes to your exercise or supplementation routines, especially if you have pre-existing health conditions.

Osteoporosis, a condition characterized by weakened bones, is a prevalent concern that significantly impacts the lives of individuals worldwide. Managing osteoporosis in daily life involves a multifaceted approach, encompassing physical health, emotional well-being, and staying informed about the latest trends in osteoporosis research. This holistic perspective is crucial for enhancing the overall quality of life for those affected by this condition.

Managing Osteoporosis In Daily Life

Osteoporosis management begins with a focus on lifestyle modifications that promote bone health and reduce the risk of fractures. Walking, jogging, and weight training are all effective ways to strengthen bones. These activities stimulate bone formation and help maintain bone density. It is essential to tailor exercise routines to individual capabilities and preferences to ensure adherence.

A balanced and nutrient-rich diet is another cornerstone of osteoporosis management. Adequate calcium and vitamin D intake are vital for bone health. Calcium-rich foods like dairy products, leafy greens, and fortified cereals, coupled with vitamin D from sunlight or supplements, contribute to maintaining bone density. Additionally, limiting excessive alcohol consumption and avoiding tobacco are integral components of a bone-healthy lifestyle.

Fall prevention is paramount for individuals with osteoporosis, as fractures resulting from falls can have severe consequences. Home safety measures, such as removing tripping hazards and installing grab bars, can minimize the risk of accidents. Regular vision check-ups and addressing issues like poor lighting contribute to creating a safe environment.

Medication adherence is crucial in managing osteoporosis. Various medications, including bisphosphonates, hormone therapy, and denosumab, aim to maintain or increase bone density. Individuals must follow their prescribed treatment plans and communicate any concerns or side effects with their healthcare providers.

CHAPTER FIVE

Coping Strategies And Emotional Well-Being

Living with osteoporosis often comes with emotional challenges, as individuals may grapple with the fear of fractures, changes in body image, and limitations in daily activities. Coping strategies are essential for maintaining emotional well-being.

Support networks play a crucial role in helping individuals cope with the emotional aspects of osteoporosis. Connecting with others who share similar experiences through support groups or online forums can provide a sense of community and understanding. Sharing concerns, fears, and successes fosters emotional resilience.

Education is empowering, and individuals with osteoporosis benefit from understanding their condition thoroughly. Learning about the disease, treatment options, and preventive measures instills a sense of control and enables informed decision-making. Healthcare providers should prioritize patient education, addressing questions and concerns to enhance patient confidence.

Counseling and mental health support can be invaluable for individuals dealing with the emotional impact of osteoporosis. Professional counseling provides a safe space to express emotions, navigate challenges, and develop coping strategies. Mental health professionals can also address issues such as anxiety and depression that may arise as a result of living with a chronic condition.

Maintaining a positive outlook is crucial for emotional well-being. Engaging in activities that bring joy, pursuing hobbies, and setting realistic goals contribute to a sense of fulfillment. Focusing on aspects of life that can be controlled and adapting to changes with resilience are key elements in fostering emotional well-being.

Future Trends In Osteoporosis Research

The field of osteoporosis research is dynamic, with ongoing efforts to advance understanding, treatment options, and preventive measures. Future trends in osteoporosis research hold promise for improved outcomes and enhanced quality of life for those affected.

Personalized medicine is emerging as a significant trend in osteoporosis research. Tailoring treatment approaches based on individual characteristics, genetics, and responses to medications allows for more effective and targeted interventions. This personalized approach aims to maximize treatment benefits while minimizing potential side effects.

Advancements in bone health monitoring technologies are poised to revolutionize osteoporosis management. From wearable devices that track physical activity and assess fall risk to advanced imaging techniques that provide detailed insights into bone structure, these innovations enable more accurate and timely assessments of bone health. Early detection and intervention can mitigate the progression of osteoporosis.

Biopharmaceutical research is seeking innovative therapy alternatives for osteoporosis. Investigational medications target particular pathways involved in bone metabolism, presenting options for patients who may not tolerate or react well to conventional therapies. The development of novel pharmaceuticals has promise for more effective and convenient solutions in the future.

Preventive techniques are gaining significance in osteoporosis research, concentrating on therapies that increase bone health before major bone loss occurs. Research in this field involves examining the influence of diet, activity, and lifestyle variables throughout various life stages to improve bone density and lower the risk of osteoporosis later in life.

Conclusion

Managing osteoporosis is a comprehensive journey that extends beyond the physical aspects of the condition. Daily life management entails a dedication to lifestyle adjustments, medication adherence, and preventative actions. Emotional well-being plays a major role, with coping methods, support networks, and a positive attitude contributing to a greater quality of life.

Looking ahead, the future of osteoporosis management is promising, with personalized medicine, technological advancements, and innovative treatments on the horizon. These developments hold the potential to revolutionize the approach to osteoporosis, offering more effective, targeted, and patient-friendly interventions.

In conclusion, a holistic and proactive approach to osteoporosis management is essential for individuals to lead fulfilling lives. By combining physical and mental well-being techniques and being updated about the newest research trends, people may traverse the difficulties of osteoporosis with resilience and positivity.